MINDFULLY MANAGING:

BIPOLAR

By Julie Knight

Practical ways to take charge of <u>your</u> life with bipolar.

Table of Contents

Introduction

Here's the scene…

*'She's curled up under the table in the kitchen, weeping and snotting and screaming at some terror that only she can see out there. This is her third day with no sleep and she hasn't got to a shower or eaten much more than a piece of toast in that time because she's been **TOO DAMN BUSY** getting her hundreds of ideas into action. Buzzing here, and buzzing there, organizing and scheduling and planning. Except no one seems to get them, dumb idiots, and they have amounted to zero anyway and sometime today she realised this and she went upstairs and slashed her arms with a razor because it was all too much…*

Nothing ever works out as she planned, and being inside her head was driving her crazy. Just crazy. Her husband is at the door, struggling to keep it quiet again for the kids and these two big men are on their hands and knees trying to coax her out, ever so gently and to get her into the ambulance that is flashing its lights at the neighbours outside, and to take her away, but she is so scared. She doesn't want to go because once she's in that place, they may never let her out again and she might never see the kids and, and, and…and these terrors layer on to the other terrors and she just wants to die…'

That's some story.

How do I know all about this?

Well, that is **my** story.

I was the woman under the table.

I was the woman with the slashed arms.

I was the woman they finally got into the ambulance and into the psychiatric hospital.

I was 42 years old and that night, in the wee small hours, a psychiatrist sat on the end of my bed and said to me

'Julie, you have bipolar. Bipolar 1.'

I knew that I had been coping with something bad since I was 17 but no-one had diagnosed me correctly or given me the right medication and support that I needed. I had already run the gamut of the fall out from suicide attempts, depressive episodes, mania and insomnia and all the self destructive behaviours that came between. As well as periods of remission which I learned not to trust.

Worse still, my family and friends had been forced to come on this journey with me, mapless and directionless, and it had not been a pleasant ride.

> **Why am I telling you this?**
>
> **Because I want you to know that I have been where you have been.**

For weeks afterwards, I felt so angry, so bitter and so completely devastated that this manic depression, as I knew it and experienced it, was real, would be with me forever and would no doubt continue to ruin my life as it already had so many times before, without end... I was labelled. I was half a person. A screw-up. I was bipolar. And I always would be.

What was the point of going on? That took a while to figure out.

But since that awful night, I **have** moved my life forward in a way that I could not have imagined. That diagnosis gave me a starting point. It drew a line under uncertainty.

I fumbled my way onwards to establish a career, something that was closed to me before, travelled, built strong and loving bonds with family and friends, and came to some kind of positive acceptance of both my bipolar and myself as a human being, worthy of love and esteem. The journey has been immensely challenging but ultimately rewarding. Right now I am not on medication. More on this later.

> *What I write about in this book is not a miracle cure for bipolar. There is not one. What it provides are practical ways to regain control of your life with bipolar. This is a lifelong process so you are in it for the long haul.*

Bipolar takes away your ability to fully control your life and to trust your decisions in a way that those without it cannot understand. You can feel rudderless and rootless.

The purpose of this book is to give you practical ways and places where you can make mindful decisions and choices and be proactive in managing your life with bipolar. I have a burning desire, and I mean a burning desire, to use my knowledge and experience to help other people with bipolar improve the quality of their lives.

These are ways that helped me get to where I am today. To be in a better place physically, mentally emotionally and spiritually. Each method is based on research, my study of psychology and the practical experiences of me and others with bipolar. Be flexible and adapt them as you need. We may all have bipolar but we are still individuals, with our own lives and needs.

That night I began to come out slowly into the light.

Come with me.

Bipolar. The facts.

Here are facts about bipolar. Just some of them.

- 1 in every 100 people has bipolar.

- It affects men and women equally.

- It is a life-long condition.

- Signs usually become obvious in the mid teens.

- The cause of bipolar is not certain. At present it seems it may be genetically based with contributing environmental factors.

- There is an increased risk of suicide if you have bipolar. Around 15% of bipolar people commit suicide. 50% will make at least one attempt to do so.

- There is an increased chance of employment instability. In the US 60% of bipolar individuals are unemployed long-term. Absenteeism is seven times higher if you have bipolar.

- Addiction to drugs and drink runs at around 56% of all bipolar people.

- Chronic insomnia is higher if you have bipolar.

- Women with bipolar are more likely to suffer from chronic post natal depression.

- Life expectancy is around 10 years less on average for bipolar individuals.

These are the facts. Unadorned and honest.

Everyone needs to know this. You and the people around you.

I am not going to make these pretty for you or write them in gentle language. This is what you and I face.

> **It is a mountain but there are ways to find footholds and climb it. Step by step.**

Chapter 1. Get diagnosed

For some of you, if you get this done, the usefulness of this book may finish right at the end of this chapter...

Before you even begin to think about anything else, get diagnosed. This may seem so intuitive as to not be worth a mention but the facts are that no one knows how many people with bipolar go undiagnosed. Moreover, results from a 2000 DMDA survey show that 69% of individuals are misdiagnosed and it takes on average 5/10 years from initial contact with a health professional for a correct diagnosis to be given.

The reasons for this are many. Bipolar can be masked or present itself as narcotic or alcohol issues, chronic insomnia, addiction to gambling or sex, a suicide attempt or, as in my case, very often it is only the depressive episodes that are actually seen by the doctor so only this is what is treated. A manic phase can be manifested in seeming schizophrenic behaviours or ADHD. It is not an easy condition to diagnose.

Sometimes it is down to us. When we feel manic we do not see any need for help or the intervention of a doctor. We are in control, impregnable and invincible. When we are severely depressed, we cannot get ourselves out of bed to clean our teeth, let alone make and keep a medical appointment. And when we are stabilised, it often seems like a horrible nightmare that we want to forget as soon as possible.

A further reason is that it is very easy to self diagnose. Bipolar was a 'disease of the week' a few years ago. Go online, look at the checklist. Tick yes and yes and yes and then we decide we are bipolar. And it is almost hip...* more on this later. Or a friend tells us we are a bit manic this week. Or we have been feeling down recently. Or a bit high. Or a family member has the condition and we think we must have inherited it. And we do not go and get it properly checked out. We are happy with our diagnosis and we are coping kind of okay... so why bother?

How do we go about taking the initial steps?

First, have a look at the checklist on the NHS UK site and see if you fulfil more than half of the criteria for both manic and depressive signs. Get a friend or family member to complete it for you and compare answers. Sorry guys, but we are not always the best judge of our behaviours!

https://www.nhs.uk/conditions/bipolar-disorder/symptoms/

While you may now be sure as a sure can be that you have bipolar, there are really good reasons for getting a professional diagnosis if you want to take the first move towards having agency in your life.

Here they are.

1. There are different types of bipolar.

   - **Bipolar 1** characterised by severe episodes of depression and mania.

- **Bipolar 2** which is characterised by milder episodes.

- **Cyclothymic disorder** where the episodes of mania and depression are brief.

- **Mixed feature disorder** where the individual may have symptoms of mania concurrent with symptoms of depression.

- **Rapid cycling** where four or more mood episodes occur within 12 months or less.

Source WebMD Medical Reference. Reviewed by Joseph Goldberg, MD July 26, 2016

You need to know which type or types that you have so you can look after yourself properly and get the best care available. These cannot be self diagnosed.

2. As stated before, we often only present ourselves to a doctor during periods of depression or are encouraged to attend an

appointment when we are in that state. I know that I first saw a doctor at 17, knowing something was badly wrong and spent 25 more years in the system, but only going to the doctor or psychiatrist when I was depressed or suicidal. This made it very hard for me or a doctor make the right diagnosis. You need a correct diagnosis to get and to manage correct interventions.

3. You may present with addiction, drug and alcohol use that is out of control and conditions such as self harm and anorexia. You need a thorough consultation to be sure that it is bipolar that you have and that these other conditions are not the actual problem but symptoms of your condition.

> 4. Most importantly, **knowledge is power.** It is not until you know what you are facing that you can start to take steps to mindfully deal with it and take control. Diagnosis is your very first step to agency.

I have already described my devastation when I was finally diagnosed with Bipolar 1. But there was also a feeling of relief. I could not always help my behaviours. I was not being a complete horror story. I could offset some of the crippling guilt. Better still, I had been given a key to hold, a key to find out more and begin to unlock doors that meant that I could move on positively.

Taking that first step is not easy.

Have a list of questions that you will want to ask the medical professional. Write them down, get the answers and note them during consultation. If you think of other questions later or you need more answers, go back and get them. Do this as many times as you need. It is your right, you need to know what you are dealing with and having the right information is an important element in regaining control of your life. This your first step towards mindful management.

I wanted to know:

- What I had.

- What the symptoms were.

- How the doctor knew this?

- What the prognosis was?

- What treatment was available?

- What medication was available?

- How quickly I could get both?

- If I could have passed it to my children?

> **If you are not happy with your initial consultation, with your relationship with your health professional or with any aspect of this diagnosis, then change your contact until you are.**

Be difficult and stubborn if you need to. You will be well practised at this… Remember the statistics on time lapsing from first consultation to final diagnosis. You want to be at the short end of these.

Take a family member or friend with you initially if you feel the need. You will probably be depressed or manic when you visit. You are not always logical or rational about your own behaviour and initial diagnosis will involve a detailed case history. If it does not, you need a new appointment. Get one.

Think about having an advocate. This is not just a family member or friend to talk about your behaviour. This is someone who understands what you want to do, and will help you speak, or speak for you if you are not able to.

And as a lifelong supporter of the UK national health system, I choke to say this, but if you can get it done more quickly privately then do. Bipolar is a killer and a fast diagnosis may save your life.

Mindful management.

1. Get diagnosed.

Chapter 2. Get medicated

Note. I am not going to write about any alternative approaches to treating bipolar that are available and may have worked well for you or someone that you know. Neither am I suggesting that these do not have a very valuable place in supporting traditional medication. I am writing from my own experience of what has worked for me. Taking medication literally saved my life.

It is really hard to know how many people with bipolar are unmedicated or receiving no treatment at all. NCBI 2010 estimate that it is probably over 50% but given the number of undiagnosed cases, the fact that there is often misdiagnosis leading to incorrect treatment being offered and the reality that those of us with bipolar often stop and start our medication at will (and you know just what I mean when I say that) then the numbers are no doubt significantly higher than supposed.

The medical term for not taking our meds is *'non compliance'*, a term that I think is absolutely terrible, carrying all sorts of negative connotations, but the most striking is the implication it carries about power differentials. We are viewed as being in a position of weakness where we must be told what to do like school children and told what is best for us. This takes our agency away. More on this kind of language later.

First, let's quickly look at why the medication we take is not always effective.

- It can be taken at the wrong time

- It can be taken in the wrong dose

- If it causes unpleasant side effects, we may avoid taking it

- It can be because there was an initial misunderstanding of what was said about dosage

- It can be because illness or pregnancy means the bipolar individual does not take it

- It can be because lack of insurance cover means the medication is too expensive

- It can be because of lack of support in ensuring there is understanding about the medication..

> **And for me, this one resonates, it can be because once we begin to feel better, we stop taking the medication, especially if it is causing side effects that are unpleasant.**

It is suggested that one in two of us do just this.

Source. www.bipolar.com

For me, I felt that I was a failure when I was taking the medications and once I felt that I was getting better, I just came off of them quietly whilst telling my partner just the opposite.

Another reason was that I **liked, loved** the start of the manic highs where you have energy, ideas and positivity. I still miss that feeling and I just felt that the medication I was on dulled my edge. And I know I am not alone in this. It was also a strange and uncomfortable feeling to perceive life like everyone else after 25 undiagnosed years of chaos, pain but also excitement and adventures. I just felt more creative and productive off the meds. More *ALIVE.*

And for a while, I was. For a while. Then the inevitable happened and my high energy spiralled into an aggressive mania followed by a terrible depression where I just wanted to die. My partner was unaware what I had been doing and mystified as to this sudden turn of events and coaxed me to a doctor where I had to front up about the fact that I had not been taking my prescription and the shock and betrayal on his face is one that I can still painfully see. Unfortunately it was not enough to stop me doing the same thing again a few months later...

So yes, I get why you do not want to be told what to take, I get your reasons for not taking medication, for being 'non compliant', but if you are going to manage your bipolar, then in my experience, you have to make the choice to do just that.

Again, this is your decision to make. You are not complying with a higher authority, **you are taking the information from the diagnosis and choosing to move forward and take control of your bipolar.**

If you had MS or chronic asthma, this is just what you would do. You would take the meds. Think of your bipolar in the same way. A long term part of your life that you have the power to manage to lessen the effects by your choices.

How to do this effectively?

1. When you get your diagnosis and the discussion turns to medication, again ask prepared questions and make notes. You have a right to know!

2. Do your research afterwards and go back and ask more questions if you need.

3. If you have side effects that are crippling, then go back and keep on going back. It may take a while to get the correct med and dose for you.

4. Again, take an advocate if you are not in a good place mentally to speak for yourself.

5. Think about how long you have had this condition and then give yourself at least half that time to recover.

6. Give them time to work. And you need to be safe and supported whilst this happens. The week I was waiting for mine to kick in after a suicide attempt was the most dangerous. I was still highly suicidal and had to be watched carefully until the effects were clear.

Once you have your meds **you must get into a routine of taking them**. Same time and place every day. This is hard for us who often live a disorganised and impulsive life. Set an alarm on your phone and have someone check in with you if you need to.

And an alarm or reminder when you are about to run short is vital. If possible, arrange for a repeat prescription to be available, for someone to call you and remind you and for someone else to be able to pick this up for you. In heavy depression, I could not make it to the bathroom to clean my teeth, let alone to the doctor to get more medication at my lowest..

And if you are missing those highs, you must think about the relapse, the side effects of these are millions of times worse than the side effects of the medication.

By taking your medication you are choosing not to just to give those around you a better quality of life, but to save your own life and to choose a life of quality for yourself.

Have a clear picture in your head of one of those times to motivate you. Or write it down if you are not a visual person. Sure, it's a horrible thing to do but it also reminds you that you have chosen to move away from this image in the best way that you can mange.

Here is mine.

I am lying in bed with cut arms and missing my children's Christmas concert because I had chosen, and it WAS my choice, to come off my medication for the third time in a year. I will never get that time back and it was not caused by my bipolar but by my choice. I was calm and in remission.

Yes, it is a guilt trip but you need to be honest with yourself! And they may well save your life...

Mindful management.

2. Get medicated.

Chapter 3. Get Eating

When you are feeling depressed or when you are manic, eating can be one of the first areas to start to go haywire. Even as you build up to a full blown manic phase, you may well feel that you do not want to eat or you forget to eat because you are too busy or too involved in your ideas. When you are depressed, your appetite may disappear, or you just cannot get yourself motivated to prepare anything.

I know from experience that it is easy for me to go all day without food for both these reasons and when I am depressed and do eat, it is often something fast, unhealthy and with limited nutritional value. Bars and bars of chocolate or hot, buttered toast are two of my choices!

You may also find that your medication causes you to lose weight, as Prozac did for me. I just found that I didn't want to eat much and lost interest in food. Or you may gain weight substantially, a common side effect of lithium and this can add yet another area to your life where you feel negative about yourself.

There is a third issue at play here as well. The major eating disorders of anorexia, binge eating and bulimia are found on average in about 2.5% of the general population of women, and the figure is around 1% for men. That is, these are the percentage of adults who will experience one or more of these disorders at least once in their lifetime.

According to a study by the University of Cincinnati College of Medicine in 2010, the comparative figure amongst people with bipolar is 14.2%, with women statistically more likely to experience one or more of the major eating disorders.

Source. https//psychcentral

That is a huge statistical difference.

The reasons were not clear to researchers. Possibly the chaotic eating caused by the bipolar became a habit, the weight gain or loss caused by medication was an issue or there is some causal link that is not clear as yet.

But this is another factor to consider when you are mindfully managing your diet. You will be more vulnerable to developing an eating disorder. If you suspect this is you, or you have such a disorder, again, professional help and advice is what is needed.

Despite many sites that will tell you otherwise, there is no obvious and replicable diet that cures or manages bipolar so what I write about here is down to common sense and my own experiences of taking control of my eating.

Have a think about your diet now.

Write down what and when you ate in the last 24 hours.

Have a go at keeping a food diary for the next week or month and see if patterns emerge.

- Are you eating regular meals? And by that I do not mean one every two days!

- Are these meals nutritionally healthy?

- Are they well balanced?

- Are there any trigger points for you in your life that mean you skip a meal or overeat?

- Are there any foods that seem to be related to changes in mood or sleep?

Certainly, my chocolate addiction caused sugar highs and then crashing lows where I became agitated and aggressive. Are there any foods that have the same effect on you?

Once you have your knowledge, here is what you need to do.

> ***You MUST eat regularly, healthily and mindfully. You must make a lifestyle change which will be with you for the rest of your life.***

This means that you need to plan ahead.

1. *Eat three meals a day.* That means no skipping breakfast.

You may need to add in a couple of snacks as well if you find your blood sugar levels collapse quickly. This is common when you are manic and burning up energy very fast.

So schedule. When and where will you eat? Set yourself half hour intervals three times everyday. And you need to stick to them, even if it means an alarm to remind you. Absolutely no excuses.

2. *The food you eat needs to be nutritionally healthy* and well balanced. You may be vegan or vegetarian or full on omnivore, but the same tenet holds true. While there is no evidence that a single diet can cure or lessen bipolar, a well balanced diet prevents swings in blood sugar, vitamin deficiency and gives you resilience for those times when you are vulnerable. There are so many sites to check out on what makes a healthy diet. I like this one.

https://www.helpguide.org/articles/healthy-eating/healthy-eating.htm

Do also check your calorific intakes are correct. You are not dieting. *You are choosing a diet that will be with you everyday and will keep you at a healthy weight.*

3. *Be prepared.* When you are stable then that is the time to get food cooked, bought or frozen ahead. Have a pile of fruit and vegetables ready to go. Make up healthy snacks ready to grab. If you cannot cook, you can make a salad, buy a healthy soup or smoothie. No excuses! Beans on wholemeal toast is one of the best balanced meals around. If you want, you can actually write up your meal plans for the week or month ahead and shop accordingly. And you can order online if you just cannot face anyone that day or that week.

4. If you have trigger foods, *then you choose if you buy them.* You have agency in this. I still have the odd bit of chocolate but I had to stop my bar a night habit!

5. Cut down or cut out the caffeine. Sorry coffee lovers! Too much will send you spinning.

6. *When you eat, do it mindfully.* If you can share your meal with someone, that is great. If not try

to eat as undistracted as you can. Again, you can choose if you sit in front of the TV or computer for every meal or not. Enjoy the taste, smell and texture of what you eat.

This continuity gives a structure to your day, gives you immunity mentally and physically against the times that you are not as resilient, lessens your chances of impulsive and unhealthy eating and it is mindful. Once again, you are choosing to control an area of your life positively. You are making a thoughtful life choice.

Mindful management.

3. Get eating.

Chapter 4. Get active

You should be seeing a theme here by now! This theme of course, is all about taking back some control of your life from a condition that often renders us chaotic and confused and with decisions about us being made by other people. We can do this in small but effective ways with lifestyle changes and one area you can manage is that of your physical activity.

Do you take any? Is it sporadic? Is it enjoyable? Is it another area where you stress?

I used to be a serial exerciser, always pushing myself to run further, lift more weights, walk harder and then getting anxious and demoralised when I failed to meet my often ridiculously unachievable goals. It was hard to keep up the kind of distances I was running when I wasn't manic and it was even harder to do anything at all when I was depressed. But I also knew that activity was working in a positive way for me when I was moderate about what I did, so when I got my diagnosis, this was one of the first areas I explored for my mindful management approach.

Research is ambivalent about whether physical activity has a serious impact on mitigating bipolar. It used to be a given that it helped, but recent studies show conflicting results and it has been proposed that in the UK health professionals should not even suggest that activity decreases depression as previously noted.

HOWEVER......

It **is** true that moderate physical activity each day releases the good old endorphins that give you a natural high, as does getting out into a green environment. This has to help with moderate depression.

If your medication is causing you to put on weight, then a little activity is going to help you with that...

It also improves your physical health and strengthens your immune system which is your armour against those times when your bipolar is worse. You can build up some extra resilience for your body to withstand some of the stresses depression and mania put upon it.

Never a bad thing.

In states of mania, it gives you somewhere to put that extra energy and allows you to focus a racing mind.

And including moderate activity in your daily routine also means that you are adding another plank to the **structure** that is your mindful management of your bipolar.

Here are a couple of provisos.

We already know that some medication can affect your weight and that some activity will aid you in managing that. But do not go crazy with the exercise. If you do, you will not keep it up everyday. This is another lifestyle change that should be long term. Sure, work out but combine it with your healthy eating.

Related to this is the fact that too much activity can lead to hypomania, so again, moderation is the key here. However manic you are feeling, you have to be mindful about the choices you make. It could be that a half marathon once a week is just what you need. But you surely do not need to do that every day!

And resist upping your targets for yourself as those of us with bipolar often do. Again, it is fine to walk a few minutes extra or swim a couple more lengths but no charts and no diaries on this one! You can do less other days as well. Do not pressurise yourself. You just do not need that in your life!

So here are guidelines.

1. You should aim to do some activity everyday. Everyday! Schedule it in as you would cleaning your teeth or your bedtime. I appreciate totally that you will not manage this with severe depression but otherwise you make the choice to get active. No excuses about the weather or the email or that drawer that needs tidying! Sure, you will let it slide at times but the overarching

aim is to include activity as a part of your every day routine.

And mentally prepare yourself that this is going to be the case for the rest of your life. See it as a positive move towards overall agency.

2. I would suggest that you **aim** for 30 minutes each day, as this is achievable and doable for most of us. You can get up a bit earlier, stay up a bit later, squeeze it in at lunchtime or take half an hour less surfing the net. Take it in chunks if you need to. Look now at your normal schedule and see where you can fit this in. If you do no activity, then just for a week add an extra five minutes a day. See how you feel and build from there.

3. Choose an activity that you enjoy or think you might enjoy. Do not go for something that is cool just now, or because you think that you should do it. I smile at my Zumba and Pilates classes. I am just not a group exerciser! Not sure what? Think back to what you loved as a child when we were all once naturally active. That will

give you a starting point. And if the first thing you try doesn't work, then shop around until you feel happy.

4. If you can, get a partner to share this time with you for extra motivation. They will encourage you on days that you just do not want to do it. You might even consider a personal trainer if you have the cash, but keep the routine simple.

5. For me, the best way to make this change was to choose an activity that was easy to do, cheap and needed little equipment. If you need to get complicated clothing and bits and pieces together, and wait for opening times and travel a long way, the chances are you will not do it regularly. For me, that has been walking. The Ancient Greeks saw walking as a form of meditation so you can add mental and emotional benefits to the physical ones. You can do this anywhere. I have done circuits of the airport concourse! You just need comfortable shoes, somewhere to walk and you are set. If you have a

green place to walk, even better. And you can walk to work, to the shops, to school with the children...But you may decide to jog, swim, cycle, lift weights...

And there is so much online that you do not have to leave your bedroom on those really bad days...

You may want to vary the shape of your activity depending on your mood. A fast, steep walk for those manic times, and a gentle stroll when you are feeling down. In times of severe depression, I have walked in the dark so I didn't have to face anyone.

Whatever you decide, make this another positive lifestyle choice. Here is my motivation to get up and walk at half past six every morning.

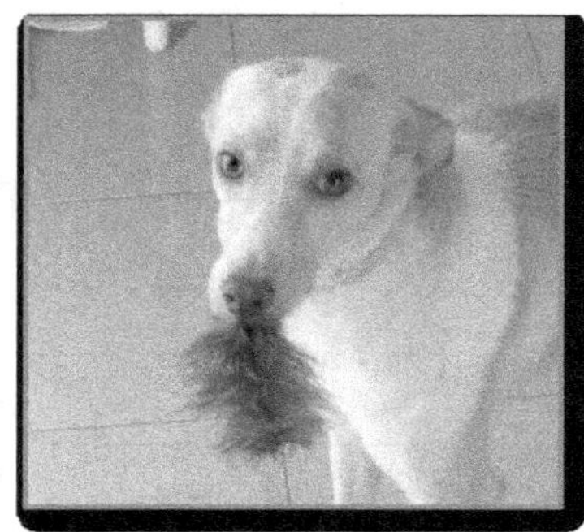

> **But the main motivation is you. You take the choice to be kind to yourself. And to give yourself the best care that you can.**

Mindful management.

4. Get active.

Chapter 5. Get rested

Getting enough sleep is an ongoing and often fruitless battle for many people with bipolar. I have spent literally my whole life fighting insomnia, tried all the suggestions from camomile tea, lavender everything, sleep hypnosis and laying in darkened rooms.

None of them work at all or at least not for long.

> **The everlasting, endless dark nights are a part of my life now and I cannot recall the last time I had a full night's sleep, even without mania and depression. Like many of you, I have had to learn to manage my life with a constant sleep deficit.**

There are two main types of insomnia. Chronic and acute. Chronic insomnia is one that occurs most nights and lasts for three months or more. Acute insomnia is one that lasts for less than a month, often caused by circumstances, but can just as debilitating. We think of insomnia as lack of sleep but it also includes hyposomnia, which is sleeping too much. The former types of insomnia seems related to manic phases and the latter to depression, so if you have bipolar you are likely to experience both types at some point in your life.

Whilst chronic insomnia affects around 4% of the general USA population, it is present in 33% of bipolar individuals. Hyposomnia is present in around 42% of the general population but is much higher if you have bipolar, at 78%.

Source. Www.ncbi.nlm.nihgv. 2014 study by CDC

Insomnia may be triggered by stress, medication side effects and also depression and mania.

Why does this matter to us? Well, if you have any experience of sleep disorder, you will know the answer to this.

Hyposomnia can affect your ability to work, to maintain relationships and to live a normal life. I clearly remember days where, whilst I did not feel severely depressed, I just wanted to shut my eyes and not go anywhere and sleep and sleep, and this could last for a week or more. Perhaps my body and mind were just saying 'Enough. I need to repair'.

Chronic insomnia affects all aspects of our health, possibly even having links to Alzheimer's onset and decreased life expectancy. However, there is a very important reason why we need to address chronic insomnia.

In 75% of bipolar individuals mania triggers this kind of insomnia. But the reverse has also been proven by recent research, something that I certainly have intuitively realised, that insomnia can actually trigger a severe dose of mania. In three quarters of us this is going to happen. I know that sometimes by around the third day of not sleeping, I just feel like I do not need to sleep ever again. My brain races, I have no need to rest or get to bed early and I can manage everything thrown at me. Or so I believe. Actually, I am getting manic. So this is a trigger factor. One that we need to monitor and address.

And I will not lie to you. I struggle with mindfully managing this area more than anything else. Once I am asleep I cannot control what my mind chooses to do, and often it chooses to wake up for the day at 2am! Then I just want to get up and get started on all of those ideas I have been laying there thinking about.

The advice below on dealing with this is based on things that have worked a little for me, for other people with bipolar that I have interviewed and are based on reading reliable research that attests to their efficacy.

1. There is some suggestion from a 2015 study on bipolar people in a manic state that **'dark therapy' can have beneficial effects,** so whilst lying in a darkened room might not make you sleep, it can reduce that spinning brain activity. It is well worth trying to sleep, or at least rest in a dark room with black out curtains and an eye mask to see if this works for you. The lack of sensory overload is a positive. If you have bipolar, then you are extra sensitive to sensory stimulation. An addition to this idea is that

weighted blankets used for autistic children can reduce feelings of restlessness and anxiety. These are not cheap but can be bought online.

2. **If you cannot sleep, then rest.** Put on an audio book or gentle music and let your body refresh itself. It needs to have a chance to heal. Bipolar puts a huge physical strain on you. If you can, and I find this very hard when I am awake in the wee small hours, do not get on to social media at all to pass the time. Sure you feel lonely and bored but put your phone in another room. Buy an alarm clock if you need to get up in the morning.

3. **Look at your diet and lifestyle.** I just never have anything that contains caffeine after 5pm. When I smoke, a couple of cigarettes throw me right off and having a day with no activity really does not suit me. So try to get active and watch the stimulants. You choose!

4. **If you can, have a siesta in the afternoon.** I live in Spain and I find the hour long rest and occasional sleep saves me! If you don't sleep at

night, it's easier to keep going and to cope if you know you can go back to bed for a siesta and even if you do not sleep in that time, then you are at least resting.

5. **Keep to a regular bedtime**, even if you do not sleep. I know that your life is often in chaos, but you do not help yourself by having irregular schedules. The odd late night is fun and doable, but these should be within the context of a routine.

6. If you really cannot sleep **then get up and do something unstimulating.** Read a book, write down a to do list for tomorrow (but do not be tempted to do any of them!), put on a gentle TV programme. Do not get into crazy planning or ideas.

7. **Have a look at meditation, breathing and yoga.** More on this later. Anything that relaxes mind, body and soul is a bonus.

7. Finally, and this is one that works for me: If you know that a few days of insomnia triggers mania, **go and get a few day's worth of sleeping**

tablets. You do not have to use them long term, but three days will give you rest and perhaps help you to restart a sleep pattern.

Mindful management.

5. Get rested.

Chapter 6. Get clean

Alcohol, drugs and bipolar go hand in hand. Do not take my word for it though. Let us look at some facts.

Alcohol use disorder or AUD, covers 11 criteria such as drinking more than planned, having to drink more than usual to get the same effects and drinking enough so that it has affected your ability to work. Fulfilling two or more of the 11 criteria over the previous year qualifies you as having AUD.

Alcohol use disorder affected 6.2% of the general population in the US in 2015.

Source. NIH 2015. National Institute on Alcohol Abuse and Alcoholism.

In people with bipolar the figure is 45%. That is a huge and significant difference.

Given that 25% of all suicides are also connected to alcohol use and the higher risk of suicide that bipolar individuals face, then it becomes of great importance in our mindful management regime to address our use of alcohol.

Source Department of Psychiatry and Behavioural Science, University of Miami. 2013.

I have been there, as one of those statistics. In fact almost from the moment my bipolar started to become apparent at around the age of 17, I turned from a rabid and evangelical non drinker to someone who just could not stop, who blacked out regularly and I continued to binge drink for most of my life. Not every day, but if I went out where there was alcohol, I just didn't seem to have an off button. I felt crap the next day. But at the time, I was on top of the world. Highly entertaining and erudite, so I appeared to myself. Actually, I was probably a complete pain in the arse! As I am sure that my husband thought as he managed the dogs and kids whilst I was tired and emotional in my bed. Again.

Do you know that feeling? 45% of you statistically will.

Let us have a look now at stats on narcotic use. This is hard to research correctly given that so many people are abusing prescribed medicines and new narcotics appear almost daily, but roughly 8.7% of the US adult population experienced NUD, narcotic use disorder, in 2014.

Source. National Survey on Drug Use and Health 2014

Guess what? You will be unsurprised to discover that the figure is much higher in those with bipolar. 41%. We are really good a coming out on top of these tables.

It gets a bit depressing, doesn't it? This is another possible area to manage and to which we are vulnerable because of our disorder. Writing thus far I am amazed that I am still here. But equally I am and so are you even though we have so much stacked against us. Be proud of that!

The research is uncertain as to what comes first. The drink, drugs or the bipolar.

However, it is clear that substance abuse disorder affects the severity of the bipolar symptoms and how likely we are to adhere to a healthy routine or to take our meds. If you are drunk you may forget to take your dosage, or if you are hungover, getting up for a brisk walk will not seem an appealing option. Equally, bipolar gives us a thin skin as far as being susceptible to developing a dependency and to relapsing. And SUD, substance use disorder, increases both our impulsivity and our depressive symptoms.

> **And we self medicate. We all do, even if we do not realise it. Often, given the prevalence of misdiagnosis and the length of time it takes to correctly diagnose the bipolar, many of us have turned to other ways to numb the pain and to cope with the day ahead. This can become a habit. Self medicating may take the guise of over eating, anorexia, self harm or developing a SUD. Or all of them.**

So what to do?

First of all, you have to take a long look at your substance use with a cold, clear eye. Is it affecting your life? Have a look at the checklist here. No lies, no cheating.

https://www.verywellmind.com/dsm-5-criteria-for-substance-use-disorders-21926

If the substance abuse is so severe that you are not functioning, you MUST GET PROFESSIONAL HELP. You cannot mindfully manage a full blown addiction.

You will be given integrated treatment. That is, the bipolar and SUD will be treated in tandem.

You make the choice to do this. Make it now. It will save your life.

Get along to AA or NA for support whilst this treatment is happening and even if it is not. There are online forums for these to help you. They will give you tools to take charge of your dependence and the help that you need.

If you are like me, and managing fairly well despite periods of binge drinking and drug taking, you still need to get clean. No drugs. No dope because it relaxes you or coke to get you up. Period.

You may need to change your friends and your lifestyle, but if you have got this far into the book, then you are already starting to do that. Keep on doing so.

Focus on getting through the next minute, the next hour, the next day. And be proud of each time you do. Replace your habits with new ones involving activity, support, mindful practices, more later and new routines.

Alcohol is a difficult one. So much of our social life in the West revolves around it, although it does seem that its use and periods of binge drinking are decreasing amongst young people aged 17/25 which may have a profound and positive effect on young bipolar people.

I went from crazy drinking to the odd binge but honestly I was not in control. I never planned to binge. But I still did and I felt awful.

I had a dose of gastritis unrelated to drink <u>while I was working in Myanmar and couldn't drink for a few months. I am now</u> 18 months into being dry despite the fact that I now live in Spain where wine is cheap and plentiful, but I just feel better for it. I have a healthy lifestyle now and do not want to binge again, and for now I just cannot trust myself not to. I suggest going dry.

If you are pressured, just say you are on medication or have an ulcer.

But, if you can get to the stage where you can take a glass or two on occasion. Do it.

Some thoughts.

You need to train yourself to think before you drink. To be mindful about the situation.

- Will this lead me to a negative place?

- Do I want this?

- Do I need another or do I just want it?

You have to be an observer. You have to be honest. You have to have control.

If you slip once, then get up and back on the horse. If you find you slip up over and over, then you need that professional help.

> **Read those statistics again. Now focus. You are going to be in the other half of the percentage. And you are going to stay there. You have choices here and you have means of support. Take them positively.**

Mindful management.

6. Get clean.

Chapter 7. Get relaxed

> **Stress is a recognised trigger for increasing symptoms of bipolar, both depressive and manic, so it is really vital that we find ways to be calm, focussed and as in control of ourselves as we can, especially as bipolar individuals have a thinner skin where stress is concerned.**

We cannot avoid stress. It comes from inside and outside. Family, career, relationships, health... and bipolar itself adds stressors to our lives, but we can explore and use methods to control the levels of stress that we feel. A useful tool for anyone!

One of the areas I really struggle with personally is my unfocussed energy. I am 56 now and should be slowing down. But even when I am not in full or pre mania, I still have lots of physical energy and a mind that seems to race with ideas, plans, thoughts and very often, worries and self doubts. This is usually 24/7 and though I can generally manage the physical side with a schedule of activity, the mental aspect has been and is an ongoing work, but I do try!

One technique I use is that I practice yoga every day of my life, even if I am tired or sick. I should say here that everyone who knows me would tell that am about as anti hippy as you can get, so please read on before you dismiss yoga as too alternative or fey for you.

Yoga is not about stretching your body into unlikely positions. It is about melding mind, body and emotions. It is about total focus and control and being kind and gentle to yourself, a valuable extra to those of us with bipolar as we are often in a place of guilt and self hatred. For perhaps twenty minutes a day you give yourself time and permission to take care of yourself, to still your mind and to reconnect.

Do not believe me? Well, there is some empirical evidence to back up my subjective experience.

A pilot study by of 70 bipolar subjects who practised yoga regularly showed that 29 reported reduced manic symptoms, and all reported increased cognitive functioning, improved mood stability and a greater adherence to their medication routine. Or more *compliance* as those who know better than us would say!

Source *newsbrown.edu*

Got to be a bonus?

You can also do yoga anywhere you can lay out a towel so if you feel bad, you do not even need to leave your bedroom. It does not cost a penny or need expensive equipment, something that makes it an easy thing to add to your life.

I use this woman.

https://yogawithadriene.com/free-yoga-videos/

The videos are free, of varied lengths and she has them for literally every situation. Yoga for when you feel down, yoga for a rainy day, yoga for self belief...Even yoga on your birthday. And there are plenty of other teachers to try if she is not your cup of tea. *'A Little Book of Yoga,'* available on Amazon has simple moves and photos for the beginner.

A couple of provisos.

Note.

- Do not get yourself into a situation where you add this activity as something you **must** do. For that reason, unless you feel strong, I suggest that you do not do any of the thirty day challenges. And you should never force yourself into shapes you don't feel comfortable with.

- Do try to do the few minutes complete relaxation at the end of each practice as it is probably us more than anyone who needs this, even if you are thinking about the next activity as you do it as I usually do!

Practice also some of the breathing videos. Alternate nostril breathing is great for giving you calm focus and stilling you racing mind.

https://yogawithadriene.com/alternate-nostril-breathing/

Other deep breathing practices give you some extra tools for when you feel stressed and wound up. Try to have one or two of these up your sleeve so that you can step away from a situation and get control of yourself and your mind and feelings again.

The 4,7,8 technique is quick to learn and easy to use.

https://www.youtube.com/watch?v=CtSRiYFbI_I

Something else that I try to do, not always successfully is meditation. An *ncbi.nlm.gov. study 2011* showed similar results to yoga for those who practised meditation regularly so I think it is safe to say that you could do one or the other for similar effects and I think the meditation takes a little less time and can be done anywhere you can sit and be quiet.

This page has a nice meditation introduction and videos.

http://how-to-meditate.org/

Again, this is about making a choice and then committing to taking control of your choices and in this way you work towards managing your bipolar.

I do have doubts that CBT can cure bipolar as has been suggested, but there may well be aspects that can be useful in your everyday approach to how you manage it, so explore areas such as ambient music, mantras and other movement based areas such as Tai Chi. These may work for you better than my suggestions. Just don't get competitive or stressed about whatever you choose!

Finally, on days when I know I am going to have extra stress or wake up feeling vulnerable, I try a little self hypnosis with a statement which I guess you could call a mantra, which varies depending on my mood. *'A Little Book of Mantras'* can help you start with this.

Those of us with bipolar are under huge strain in all areas of our beings and choosing one or two of these short activities can really be a gentle act of kindness to ourselves.

Mindful management.

7. Get relaxed.

Chapter 8. Get trigger happy

One of the most vital skills that you will need to learn and to practice to manage your bipolar mindfully is to be able to identify and avoid potential triggers. Triggers are something that seem to set off a manic or depressive episode. Triggers are not the only cause of a polar episode but they certainly can play a part.

It can be really hard to identify your own triggers objectively, especially if they are ones that you enjoy, and you may want to ask a family member or friend of they have any pointers on this. What have they noticed that can trigger you into a period of depression or mania?

Also be aware that certainly for me and I am sure for you there may be different triggers for depression and mania. Unless it is a reaction to a situation, I find depression can literally come out of a clear blue sky, although I sometimes notice that I have wanted to sleep and eat more for a day or two before, whereas for mania without a doubt it is a run of not sleeping that can cause this, as for me can certain drugs and overloading on sensory stimulation, for instance listening to certain types of music over and over again.

One common trigger for either end of the polarities has been identified as stress. This is true for 100% of people with bipolar

Source. Journal of Affective Disorder. 2014.

We discussed stress in the previous chapter, and you absolutely must be vigilant about reducing stress as far as possible in your life, both externally in terms of work and relationships, and internally by managing your levels yourself. You cannot avoid stress caused by death, unemployment and so on, so you have to manage those areas that you can.

Another potential trigger for us is having a baby. Women who have bipolar are 40|% more likely to develop a postpartum depression than those who do not have the condition. I did. Twice.

Source

https://www.postpartumdepression.org/resources/statistics/

I am not advocating you never have kids but you should be aware that PND, or post natal depression is a higher risk for you, so you need to have plans in place to manage this and to make sure medical practitioners involved in your pregnancy and the birth are aware of your condition from the outset. This is especially important as you may need to change your medication during pregnancy and whilst you are breast feeding.

Drugs and alcohol are potential triggers for many of us as we have already seen, as is lack of sleep or a period of sleep disruption. For this reason jet-lag can be a trigger. This site has some good facts and tips for you.

Source.

mania.https://blogs.psychcentral.com/bipolar-laid-bare/2017/08/jet-lag-bipolar-disorder

Another trigger which I only just realised as I was typing this is lack of sunlight. I am having my first winter back in Europe after four sunny years in Asia and I am struggling. As the days are getting greyer, I am getting lower and lower and having to work to keep active and eat well. Whilst there is no definitive link between SAD, seasonal affective disorder, and bipolar, some of us are certainly aware of our moods changing with the seasons. For these winter blues, vitamin D, light therapy and melatonin are options. I prefer the idea of two months in Thailand but I guess the vitamins are cheaper...

Social media can be a trigger in two major ways. Firstly, comparisons of your life with others can cause depression and the actual act of being online for long periods can trigger mania, especially if you get up and turn on the phone when you cannot sleep. And it is easy to go on an online gambling or shopping binge. Getting into a place where you are constantly reading about your condition can be helpful but can also take you dark places. Unless you are checking out a specific fact or site, steer clear of the wormhole. You know the facts. They are horrible. Do you need to keep revisiting them? Is it helpful? No!

OK. Those are general triggers and you may have already identified some of these that have meaning for you. Let us get focussed now. It is helpful knowing what your own triggers, are but managing them mindfully is a little more challenging.

Once you have identified your general triggers, you have to be completely mindful and vigilant about spotting them.

For instance, I found that if I went out drinking early in the evening just for one or two after work, I would still be there at midnight, completely drunk, throwing out my sleeping, eating and every other calming activity and that this could then be the start of mania. I have had to make the conscious decision to take one of two options. If I am asked to go out, I can either refuse with a white lie if I need, or I can set myself the goal of leaving after one drink. For me, the former is the wise choice. I know that I cannot manage the latter.

If I know that four sleepless nights cause me to go into a manic episode I go and get medication. This is prearranged with my GP. You may need to do the same.

It may be that a specific circumstance such as flying abroad is a trigger for you. Be prepared and plan ahead for this.

> **And hard though it may seem, you may have to review the circumstances of your life in some ways.**
>
> **It may mean changing your job if you can, it may mean ending a relationship or dropping friends who are unhealthy for you. These are difficult and painful choices but if they balance your mental health, you must take them.**

This has meant for me avoiding or cutting out certain people from my life. People who cause me stress and negativity, people whom I seem to behave in a negative way towards, people who try to get me into competitive situations or those who drink, party or keep me up to late. Actually, let's be real here. I keep **myself** up too late. It is my choice to do this. This is no judgement on them. They can do all this and function, as people who have god mental health can. But these are not folk that it is healthy for me to be around. I have found it better to have a few friends around me rather than lots, and I accept this.

Try not to set yourself rigid goals in any aspect of your life as these just add stress, whether it be getting a promotion, how many steps you walk that day, how many calories you consume. Add goals that are general and positive. I will do a little physical activity today, I will eat breakfast, I will take time to sit and enjoy the view or to do my deep breathing…. Anything with numbers or times involved is a likely trigger for stress.

You have no choice about your bipolar but you do have choice over avoiding or mitigating trigger situations, substances or people. Yes, you do! And you need to be hyper aware and make the healthy choice for yourself.

This will take supreme effort of will. And will is something we lack at certain times of our bipolar journey, so use remission to set strong habits. There's no easy way to sugar coat this pill but all I can say is that eventually it will become easier and second nature. You are aiming to make these a natural and integral part of your life.

Mindful management.

8. Get trigger happy.

Chapter 9. Get supported

Bipolar can make you feel as if you are living in a lonely and bleak landscape. No one else really understands what it is like to be inside your head, what your depression, your mania and your guilt feel like. Even you and I will have very different experiences of bipolar. And it is easy to isolate ourselves, to go into our own little space, one that we can control, where we do not have the extra stress of social engagement and where we can be alone to cope as best we can. I have just retreated sometimes. It is easier than explaining.

Do not do this. Or at least, do not make this your default position. Get support just as you would if you had long term diabetes, MS or a chronic heart condition.

A report from the Bipolar Wellness Centre reveals that those of us who have some support show decreased depression, more stable moods and recover from the polarities more quickly than those who do not. And it also shows that strong relationships help us cope better with bipolar on a daily basis.

When I was first diagnosed, I was very reluctant to get medical help or to share my experiences of bipolar with people around me. Indeed, as I wrote earlier, this book will come as a surprise and a shock to some people who have known me for decades, and I am editing this feeling nervous about 'going live', so to speak.

I always felt that I should be able to cope alone. I was educated, I had a degree in Psychology and worked successfully in social care with children from a background of deprivation. I had coped for many years. Just. Actually, not coped. I had somehow survived situations and behaviours that actually scare me now to think about.

I also thought that people would judge me. And let us not fool ourselves. Whilst good work is being done in this area, there is a still a stigma attached to what is perceived as any mental illness. We are judged.

But I found that even a little help really did help! After my diagnosis, I was angry, bitter and resentful at the wasted time, life and opportunities, but once I started to explore the options for my future, my own situation and that of those close to me improved. This was not a magic wand moment, but a gradual clearing of the smoke. So do not be proud. Get the support that you deserve! Make that choice!

The Bipolar Wellness Centre identifies two types of useful support. Social and informational. I hadn't thought of them like this before, but it is a really useful definition.

Here are what I have found has helped me in both arenas, social and informational.

6. ***Medical practitioners.*** These come in many guises, including your psychiatrist, your GP and your therapist...but it is up to you to use each one in a way that helps you. There is no shame in this. These are experts in their area just as your mechanic or your plumber is and they can help you directly and/or refer you on for

additional assistance as required. And from each get as much information as you can. I know I am fortunate to have been treated in the NHS in the UK and for those of you who have to pay, it is more difficult, but within constraints, get that medical care. You have a condition. You need it. Reread the chapter on getting diagnosed. My GP admitted she had no knowledge of bipolar but moved heaven and earth to find out what I needed and to see me through the first weeks until medication took hold.

5. *Advocates.* You will not always be capable of expressing what you need. Not because you are inarticulate, but because the bipolar can take the words away. If you have a significant other who can advocate for you in the medical centre, the bank, work, then use them.

I could sometimes croak to my husband what I needed and he could speak for me at the surgery while I sat mute and weeping. Or you can write it down and hand it over to your advocate. If you don't want to or can't use a family member or friend as an advocate. Explore whether you can be provided with an advocate through mental health services or a charity. And on this front, consider if someone needs to be given power of attorney in case you cannot manage your finances.

The Bipolar Support Network UK can give advice on this and the related topic below. There is a Facebook page.

4. **Work.** Establish a strong relationship with the appropriate person at work. These may be in HR or through a union. All you tell them is confidential and I found this really helped me. I worked in a school and the school nurse became the person I spoke to. Perhaps you may need to work at home sometimes or take time off for medical attention. Can you arrange flexitime for this? Can your contact do this?

3. **Family.** This can be a double edged sword. For some of us, family has been an exacerbating factor in our bipolar, so you need to fit this group to your circumstances. This may be a

definite no for you. If you have one or two close family members whom you trust, then share with them, ask them to help you with triggers, child care, regular support and check ins. You would do the same for them. My sister has been a great support to me, by doing little obviously, but I know that she knows and that is often enough!

This person may be your partner, and if you are in a long term relationship with someone, they will often fulfil many roles. Advocate, carer, child care....This can really strain your relationship so others in this role help hugely to take some of the pressure from you both.

2. *Friends.* Very few of my friends know more than my surface details about bipolar and many of them who read this will be shocked at the depth of my condition, even though they have known me for 25 years. This is due to my pride and my English hatred of worrying anyone. But I am not sure this has been very useful for me! The younger generation seem to be more open

about sharing and caring and a couple of good, supportive friends to help you out are essential! So on this one, its do as I say, not as I do!

> **1. And the very best support that you can have is *yourself.* Find out all the information that you can, make choices that are healthy and positive for you. Be very kind to yourself. Be mindful about your bipolar, the choices you make to manage it and the relationships that you develop. You need people around you whom are supportive, knowledgeable and there for the long haul. Bipolar takes a huge toll on relationships. Cherish and nurture them in those times that you are in balance and nurture and cherish yourself too.**

Finally, ask those involved with you to read about bipolar and share information with them. Do not cut them out of the loop. You may consider group, parenting or relationship therapy to help you all.

Those close to you will feel concern, guilt, worry and stress too. But equally, they have chosen to be with you whatever and you should acknowledge and value that wonderful gift. It also means that they see something valuable and wonderful in you!

Mindful management.

9. Get supported

Chapter 10. Get real

Here is a list of famous people with bipolar.

- Beethoven

- Ernest Hemingway

- Van Gogh

- Lincoln

- Mozart

- Newton

- Churchill

What a group to be part of! You too are one of these geniuses, these giants of creativity and knowledge. You are part of an elite. That's something to cling to in dark times, isn't it? We have all looked at these names and perhaps felt a little better, a little more cosy in our condition.

OK. Let us get real here. The romanticising of bipolar is not helpful to me or to you. And as a youngster I just revelled and indulged myself in the romantic pain of being mentally ill, clutching my Sylvia Plath poems close, even before I knew what I had. I knew I was destined to be a tortured writer and artist, albeit one who was usually too ill to actually write. And when I did, it wasn't quite as wonderful as I had hoped. It didn't feel so romantic when I was face down on my bed weeping but hey, that's all part of the genius game! Nonsense.

First of all, is your name on that list? No. Is it ever likely to be on that list? Probably not.

Secondly, none of these people was actually diagnosed medically with bipolar. These are suppositions made from reported behaviour. These names have become a lazy shorthand for the supposed link between creative genius and bipolar.

Thirdly, even if these people did have bipolar, and we know that there are many famous people diagnosed and visible in the media who do have the condition, do not believe for one moment that their life was any less painful, difficult and challenging than yours, and they lived in times where treatment was basic and mental hospitals as they were known were places of horror and despair. Churchill did not talk about the Black Dog on his shoulder to just to be poetic. He was describing a very real emotion that limited his life.

Dissuade yourself from this view of your bipolar.

Equally, it has not been helpful to us when bipolar has been, and probably will be in the future, a 'disease of the month.' It is great that celebrities and professionals are bringing it to public awareness, but again, do not fool yourself that what you have is hip and trendy and makes you cool. This spurious sheen of coolness has led to people actually asking to be diagnosed with bipolar. *ASKING TO BE DIAGNOSED WITH BIPOLAR?!* This, from a BBC news report in 2010.

> *'A new diagnosis of bipolar disorder might also reflect a person's aspiration for higher social status and a feeling that by having the condition they too are creative.'*

Do not buy into this idea that having bipolar means you are super creative or a genius of some sort. Perhaps you are. But bipolar and all of these characteristics do not correlate as neatly as some researchers would like us to believe. If you start to believe this kind of evidence is true, then you are less likely to want to manage the bipolar, and do not let anyone else tell you otherwise. It may be entertaining and amusing for some people around you to see you manic and high. You are not here to be entertainment for anyone. It is a real issue for you and they need to be told just that. So reclaim your power.

What you have is lifelong and, at present, incurable. You need to accept that and take the long view of your own care. You need to look short, medium and long term at what your goals and needs are and you need to be clear eyed and honest about that.

> **It is very easy with bipolar to become pliant, to believe that you have no free will or self control over what you do, that others know best what you need and that this condition will always be in charge of your life. Equally, it is very easy to take the opposite view. That no one understands what you are going through, and so cannot possibly help you.**

Twist these ideas straight on their heads.

There are plenty of times when you are in remission when the reverse is true. Plenty of days and hours where you manage. Focus and build on those times and all the times that you have walked through the fire and come out the other side. Focus too on the fact that you have been far out to extremes that many other people never experience and turn the pity for yourself to compassion and help for others.

Take charge of the vocabulary surrounding your bipolar. I choose not to see or refer to myself as a sufferer, as being non compliant, as being mental or as having a disease and I have deliberately tried to avoid using that vocabulary throughout this book. I prefer language that permits control, volition and remission into my life. I like words such as 'living with' or 'having a disorder' in just the same way as someone with ME or MS is living with a condition.

Use the **language of managment** as you speak and educate others to do the same. Interestingly there is a strong movement in medical and self help circles for just this approach. You choose the words that mean something powerful to you when talking about bipolar and that give you strength. They may be different from mine. That's just fine. Sometimes I have used manic and depressed, because that is exactly how I feel and I find 'bipolar' just doesn't get close to what I am dealing with!

When you are first diagnosed, it is really easy to slide into the kind of mindset that says **I am bipolar**. As if this is your entirety. No you are not. You are a husband, a son, a mother, a worker, a friend, a writer, a runner, a cook, a reader, a dreamer, a lover...who has the condition of bipolar.

> **If you see bipolar as your first and foremost defining characteristic then you will filter your view of yourself and the view of others about you through that lens, so define yourself in all of your strength based roles first.**

See yourself as a work in progress. Just like everyone else around you. Set yourself positive goals and ambitions. Take pride in the fact that you have come this far and plan how much further that you are going to go. Because by taking mindful control of your bipolar, by using thoughtful management and taking healthy choices as outlined above that is what will happen.

A couple of small things to end with.

Be kind to yourself. Everyday.

Be understanding of yourself. Everyday.

Be the best that you can be. Everyday.

Take control, be mindful, be alive. Everyday.

I send you love and respect for what has gone before and what is to come.

Mindful Management

10. Get real

End note

You might not find <u>all</u> of these ideas helpful, and they are certainly not all easy to carry out, day in and day out for a long time. I live it. I know it! And you are still going to get times where it all seems too much!

Utilize each tool as often as you need it. They are there for you to choose and use.

I got up this morning feeling bleakness in my heart and the lure of just going back to bed and hiding was strong! But I got through the first hour of by having breakfast, ignoring my emails until I felt stronger and doing a little yoga and then I could manage to face the rest of the day. **I had to make the decision to do this and you have to make the decisions too,** and this is one area where you can have control, not be controlled.

So seize the opportunity! You have that power to change and to influence how your next hour goes and then the next...

Here I am later on that day.

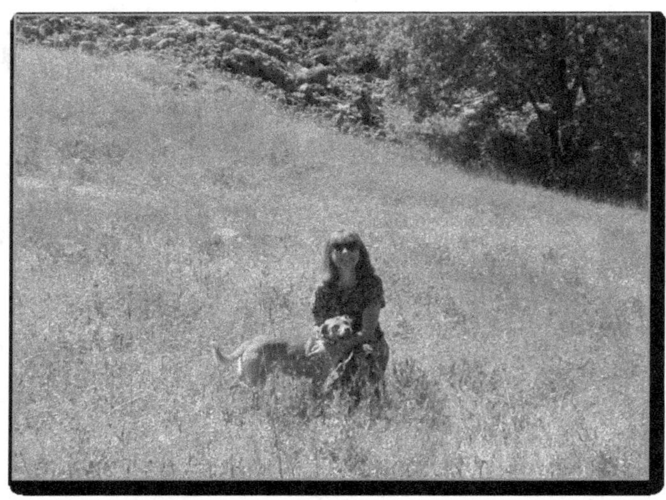

Tomorrow? Who knows but for now, **I** am I am in the driver's seat.

Contact Me

If you need more help in mindfully managing your bipolar or in talking about any of the issues that this book has raised for you, then leave feedback and share your own experiences on the forum where you bought this book. Our support for each other is another area of strength in our mindful management of bipolar.

I also offer bespoke bipolar support sessions, tailored to suit your needs.

I have been where you are right now and can help you to positively move forward with your life.

Please mail me at **BEElieve** here for this.

greyqueenbee@gmail.com

Thank you.

About the author

Julie Knight is a freelance writer and English teacher. She was born and raised in beautiful Sussex, UK and this gave her a love of the countryside and walking. She later spent twenty years in the Scottish Highlands with her children and a revolving menagerie of furry creatures. Over the years she has had a career in social work, caring for children with emotional and learning issues and as a teacher of English in countries as diverse as Italy and Myanmar.

She is now located in Andalusia, Spain with her husband and enjoys the relaxed lifestyle, fostering dogs and hiking in the hills around the town. More travel is on the cards....

She was diagnosed with bipolar 1 at the grand old age of 42...

A BEElieve book for QUEENbee Publications

Disclaimer

This book provides advice and guidance on dealing with bipolar disorder drawn from personal experience and research. It is not intended as a substitute for professional advice, diagnosis, or treatment. Always seek the advice of your doctor or other qualified healthcare provider with any questions you may have regarding your mental or physical wellbeing or a medical condition. Do not disregard professional medical advice or delay in seeking it because of anything you may read in this book.

The author and publisher accept no liability for any injury arising out of the use of material contained herein, and make no warranty, express or implied, with respect to the contents of this publication.